How to Avoid the Medical Tiger Trap and

GET YOUR LIFE BACK

How to Avoid the Medical Tiger Trap

and Get Your Life Back

DR. MELODIE BILLIOT

*A tiger trap is a deep
hole covered over with
grass that you can't see
until after you have
fallen into it.*

CONTENTS

FOREWORD

"I am calling about your biopsy pathology report. The doctor wants you to come in as soon as possible for a consultation."

I was a 27-year-old newlywed. Two years earlier I had graduated with my doctorate as valedictorian of my class, bought my own practice, and had just bought my first house. I had thought I was on top of the world.

This was to be my personal lesson in how a serious health problem can change your life.

I spent the next week stressing out while researching and calling multiple doctors for more information. It was amazing how little real help was available to me. Every doctor I talked to gave me the same advice:

"Based on your diagnosis, you must have surgery, which may leave you sterile."

When I suggested any other course of action to try to get my body to heal without surgery, I was told, somewhat condescendingly, that that wasn't possible. When I wanted some time to try to research non-surgical solutions, I was threatened and finally dismissed from my doctor's care.

This is a story of my own full recovery (yes, I have two wonderful sons, now) and how what I learned from my experience has since changed the lives of many thousands of my patients.

This book is a summary of my own experience—added to my 20+ years spent helping patients with serious health problems to recover their health.

> **If you have a difficult health problem, what I can teach you in this book could change your life.**

TEN CLUES THAT YOUR HEALTH MAY NEED SERIOUS ATTENTION

When I look back at my own health prior to my diagnosis, it's apparent in hindsight that I had set myself up to have a health problem. Years of school stress, a terrible diet and lots of sugary foods had damaged my health, but I justified all my symptoms—"Everyone has these problems." "It's not all that serious." "It's not keeping me from going to work."... and so on.

I have since realized that the best advice for my patients is to face up to the realities of their health conditions and stop any minimizing and a *covering-it-all-up* attitude. Had I done this early on, I might have avoided a lot of misery.

How many of these ten clues do you find yourself experiencing? (Be honest with yourself!)

1. Your symptoms are getting in the way of your life, with problems such as *pain, fatigue, insomnia, brain fog,*

depression, menstrual and menopause problems, allergies, irritability, weight gain, anxiety, gas, bloating, reflux, indigestion, constipation, diarrhea, breathing problems, low immune response, rashes, joint pain, vision and hearing problems, itchy skin, hair loss, acne, back pain, neck pain, headaches, infertility, low libido, trouble concentrating, memory problems, sugar cravings, bone loss, blood sugar problems, high blood pressure, heart problems, high cholesterol and many more.

2. Doctors and treatments that you try don't help or resolve these symptoms and leave you angry, sad or frustrated.

3. Doctors or others say or imply that there's really nothing wrong with you, maybe "it's all in your head," or that you're getting all the treatment available, so why are you still whining? This despite obvious (to you) serious health problems you are experiencing.

4. You feel like your spouse, boss, coworkers and friends have no clue that you just aren't functioning normally a lot of the time.

5. You feel frustration, disappointment and guilt that you can't keep up with everything. Or, you are paying a

physical and mental price just to do the minimum required in your life.

6. You are upset by the money you have wasted in co-pays, uninsured medical treatment and drugs, therapies and the 50 bottles of vitamins on your shelf that didn't work.

7. You feel like you are missing out on your life—with periods of time you aren't fully "there" to participate and experience. You've lost opportunities with family and friends that you had to turn down because you just weren't up to it.

8. You are confused by all the conflicting information on the Internet and in books about why you might have your problems and what would work to make them go away. And you feel frustration at all the "other people" who say these things helped them... when they aren't helping you.

9. You have a recurring fear that you never will find a solution and that the rest of your life is going to be this way.

10. You have a recurring fear that what is going on with you now is going to get a lot worse in the future.

If you have a number of these "clues," know this:

> **Based on interviewing tens of thousands of patients with these issues, almost none of them had ever resolved their health problems.**

Here is why they failed:

The information you've relied on most of your life about health care isn't strictly true.

If you're like most people with stubborn health issues, you will try several ways to reduce your problems, such as drugs, vitamins, exercise, restricting your diet, etc. Some of these may work for a time to make your problems less awful. But the overwhelming odds are that nothing you try will permanently heal your problems (in fact, you may have been told—and believe—that there is no resolution for your problems).

You, along with everyone else in the US have had a lifetime of exposure to our current health care system. Because of this, the information you have been given and may "know to be true" about your problems and how to treat them is based on a system that fails to effectively treat chronic health problems. Further, the healthcare system operates with arrogance:

This attitude tends to discourage anyone from looking beyond the traditional system when it fails and can prevent you from finding a solution that works.

This faith in medicine is very deep-rooted.

I have often had patients that "relapsed" into medical care because they simply got afraid that "just" helping their body to heal itself using natural methods was insufficient, and that they needed to be "more proactive, more aggressive" with their problem. In almost every case, they returned to my office disillusioned (again) with medicine—and in worse condition.

This almost happened to me when my first child developed severe allergies at the age of two months. Over a period of about a week, he went from being a normal, healthy baby to being covered with a weepy rash and vomiting up everything I fed him, including breast milk. Nothing I knew or tried helped at all. He just got worse, with projectile diarrhea added to the vomiting. His weight began to fall, and at age six months I had to take him to the hospital to handle severe dehydration.

At the hospital, the doctors diagnosed him as "failure to thrive" but could find no cause. They dismissed the idea of allergies, and ordered a feeding tube and referrals to various specialists for experimental testing.

I was torn. They seemed so confident, even though they admitted they had no answers at all. I seriously considered putting myself and my baby in their hands and "going the medical route." It made so much sense! They had so much training, so much technology, equipment, big buildings, and my whole family was in complete agreement that this would be the "best way to go." I was terrified that my baby would die; I wanted someone to save him!

Fortunately, all my years training in science saved me. I asked myself, "What part of 'we have no answers' do I not understand?" Then I assessed what I *did* know and realized that I understood a lot about my son's problems, where they came from, and even a direction to go toward helping his body heal. The medical doctors had zip, zero, nada—no definite answers, just "experimental testing." This was an easy decision; it just required me to be willing to take full responsibility and completely buck the general agreement of the whole society (and my family).

I ignored the warnings—dire warnings—and finally, threats of child services action, and I took my son out of the hospital. He was losing weight daily, headed for birth weight, so to say the least, we needed a solution in a big hurry.

I mobilized my friends, some of the best holistic practitioners and researchers in the country. They all joined the fight to save my son. My husband took the baby to Florida to work with a doctor who tested him and discovered a formula that would sometimes stay down and he began to gain weight. The doctor used a technique to desensitize my son to this formula that made a huge difference in his body accepting it. Shortly afterwards, I went to Los Angeles to train under Dr. Devi Nambudripad (the doctor credited with discovering allergy elimination techniques) and learned acupressure therapies to desensitize food allergies. My husband left Florida and took the baby to upstate New York to work with two phenomenal nutrition doctors to help heal his digestion issues.

I then started him on a regimen of acupressure and nutrition, which over a period of three years, resulted in a healthy, normal child.

What a learning experience that was!

So, when a patient feels they must "go the medical route," I really, *really* understand. Of course, some problems truly are medical problems. These issues can be expected to resolve with medical treatment, and sometimes the side effects of the treatment are acceptable. Broken bones, severe infections, and diseases requiring body systems support all fall into this category.

But the average person has absolutely no idea what can be accomplished with **modern non-medical technology working with the body to help it to heal itself.** In fact, most are not even looking for non-medical solutions.

This is because there is a very, very important fact they haven't yet discovered:

There are little to no effective medical treatments for the resolution of chronic health problems—but almost no one is talking about this.

In fact, the most common way people discover this fact is by being told by their doctor that there is "nothing more that can be done for you." You developed a problem and dutifully went to your doctor to have it fixed—fully expecting a cure or a resolution, some answer or resolution for your problem. Then, suddenly, you are stuck with your problem with no solution, no answers at all.

THE TIGER TRAP OF MODERN MEDICAL CARE

> **A tiger trap is a deep hole covered over with grass that you can't see until after you have fallen into it.**

Chronic health problems are those that recur regularly or never go away. These make up a huge majority of all health problems (seventy-five cents of every health care dollar).[1] The gaping, but camouflaged hole in modern health care is that there are almost no solutions for these problems, only drug management to make some of the symptoms more tolerable:

- Diabetes: (20+ million) insulin for the rest of your life keeps you comfortable...until you begin to lose extremities and have kidney or heart failure.

- Hypothyroidism: (30+ million) a lifetime drug use will fix your lab values while rarely helping your symptoms, leaving you with little energy, brain fog and anxiety, weight gain, digestive distress and little interest in life.

- High blood pressure: (75+ million...1 in 3 adults) drugs for the rest of your life have devastating side effects, leading millions to quit taking them. In fact, only fifty percent of patients diagnosed have their condition under control with the drugs. This leads to heart attacks, stroke and kidney failure.

This massive omission is not discussed or pointed out publicly; indeed, you may be completely unaware of it yourself... until you develop this type of problem and find yourself looking up from the bottom of the tiger trap with no way out.

Before you developed a chronic condition, chances are you had the same ideas that most of the unaffected population does:

"What's a chronic health condition?" "If you are sick, just go to the doctor—what's the big deal?"

This is reflected in the media's reporting on health care, which consists of politics, business, medical and drug studies that make the news and current events. Nowhere is it pointed out that nearly half of the public reading the news has a health problem with no effective treatment available.

What the media and public are not noticing is the individual suffering from long-term chronic health conditions. This suffering reduces happiness and productivity for them and their families. These are not the severely ill who are bedridden, living on disability or requiring constant care. **They are the "walking ill,"** people who hold down jobs, take care of their families, raise children and are active in churches and other organizations. But every day they wonder if they can keep it up. They're battling fatigue, depression, pain, brain fog and the conviction that it's all likely to get worse. They believe this because over many years of searching and effort, they have found no effective treatments or solutions. These people have found that medical technology is very close to bankrupt about chronic illness, other than temporary or long-term drug management of symptoms.

"You are healthy, congratulations!"

The nature of many chronic health problems is that sometimes they don't show as out of range on blood tests or as anything of concern during a standard physical. The person will complain of many symptoms to their doctor, but the doctor may tell them they are perfectly healthy (by lab results and examination). They may be told to reduce their stress, eat less fat and get more rest, but there is no diagnosis to be made. Often if the person continues to insist that there is something wrong, the doctor will suggest, "It's possibly depression or a 'stress-related' issue," (inferring that if the doctor fails to find the problem, it must be because the patient is making it up— "it's just in your head"). Often patients are prescribed an anti-depressant or other psychotropic drug.

> **Half the US population has one or more chronic health condition.**

If you have chronic problems yourself, be aware that this is much, much more common than you might imagine. According to the CDC, about half the US population (133 million) has one or more chronic health conditions and one in four has two or more conditions. The CDC reports that 7 out of the top 10 causes of death are chronic diseases.[2]

To illustrate with just a single condition, arthritis causes more than 22 million Americans to have trouble with their usual activities (CDC).[3] Modern medicine has no cure for arthritis and can only "manage" it if possible with drugs, all with severe side effects* (see below for examples). Further, there is no arthritis case that has *only* arthritis. This is a condition of chronic inflammation, which creates a host of other chronic health problems to go along with the debilitating joint pain.

***Side effects of arthritis drugs:**

NSAIDs: Blood clots, heart attack, stroke, liver damage, damage to gut lining leading to "leaky gut."

STEROIDS: Cataracts, bone loss, increased blood sugar and appetite.

DMARDs: Increased susceptibility to infection.

BIOLOGICS: Increased risk of serious infections.[4]

> ***If you have fallen into this camouflaged hole, this Tiger Trap, don't be fooled into imagining that anyone is coming to your rescue.***

There are no miracle cures "right around the corner" because the health care system is completely stuck on the **drug treatment model,** which does not work for most chronic problems.

David Shaywitz, a health care reporter writing in *Forbes* magazine inadvertently got it right. In an article defending the pharmaceutical industry from charges of withholding "cures they don't want you to know about" he writes:

> *"The unfortunate truth is that drug companies really want to cure disease, but rarely know how. Medical science simply isn't up to the challenge. Most diseases aren't well enough understood to enable the rational development of truly transformative treatments."*[5]
>
> **-David Shaywitz, *Forbes* magazine**

Of course, by "treatments" Mr. Shaywitz means "drugs." A drug is a chemical that forces the body to react, not a resource that the body can use to heal itself from a chronic problem. There may be no conspiracy to keep the cure for your problems hidden, but the truth is just as bad: **Most of the research being done to treat chronic problems is in drugs, which are not, and never have been, an effective solution.**

To sum up:

- There is a class of health problems that can ruin (or is currently ruining) your health, life and happiness, and affects at least 50% of the US population.

- There is little to no effective medical treatment available if this happens, or has already happened, to you or your family.

- There is little understanding or empathy for these sufferers, as most of the world seems to believe that doctors know how to treat all but the "big name" (cancer, MS, Alzheimer's, etc.) diseases quite effectively. If you are suffering from other than a "big name" disease and are whining about it, the popular thinking is that you need to go get treatment and, frankly, suck it up. You don't have a REAL problem. In some cases, this attitude may be shared by your doctor.

THE CHRONIC HEALTH CONDITION

There are two kinds of health problems:

First, there is what I would term a "medical problem," where the symptom itself is the problem. If your arm is broken, the symptom is a broken arm—which is also the problem. A medical doctor would successfully treat the symptom, which would also fix the problem. There are thousands of examples of this type of problem, from appendicitis to trauma.

The second type of problem is called a "chronic condition" by medical doctors. This is an ongoing problem, which keeps recurring or never goes away (such as high blood pressure, diabetes, heart disease, arthritis, chronic fatigue, depression, anxiety, etc.).

Chronic health problems are caused by a compromise in the body's ability to maintain and heal itself.

Medical doctors can't, and don't, treat the causes of chronic conditions, just the symptoms. Treating these symptoms can be a very good thing, such as drugs to reduce high blood pressure and prevent stroke. But if this is the only solution, and the patient must take the drugs (with side effects and stress to the body) for the rest of their lives, then this isn't such a good solution at all.

ORIGINS OF CHRONIC HEALTH CONDITIONS

Bad news: You live on Planet Earth. Therefore, you'll have damage to your body repeatedly as an inevitable result of living. Your body will repair the major damage, but if your ability to heal is compromised, some of the damage, a "tag-end," is often left *permanently unrepaired.* The body arranges a work-around to maintain its function despite these unrepaired "tag ends" but this results in a permanent area of stress.

Your body is designed to hide the symptoms of stress if it possibly can, so at first you may be unaware of any problem. Over time, more stress builds from repeated incomplete repairs until the body can't control it—and you become aware of a symptom. Notably, a symptom from this source generally won't go away once it begins. There is no medical solution available other than to treat the symptom itself, as it is caused by long-term stress from many areas of unrepaired damage, none of which is medically treatable.

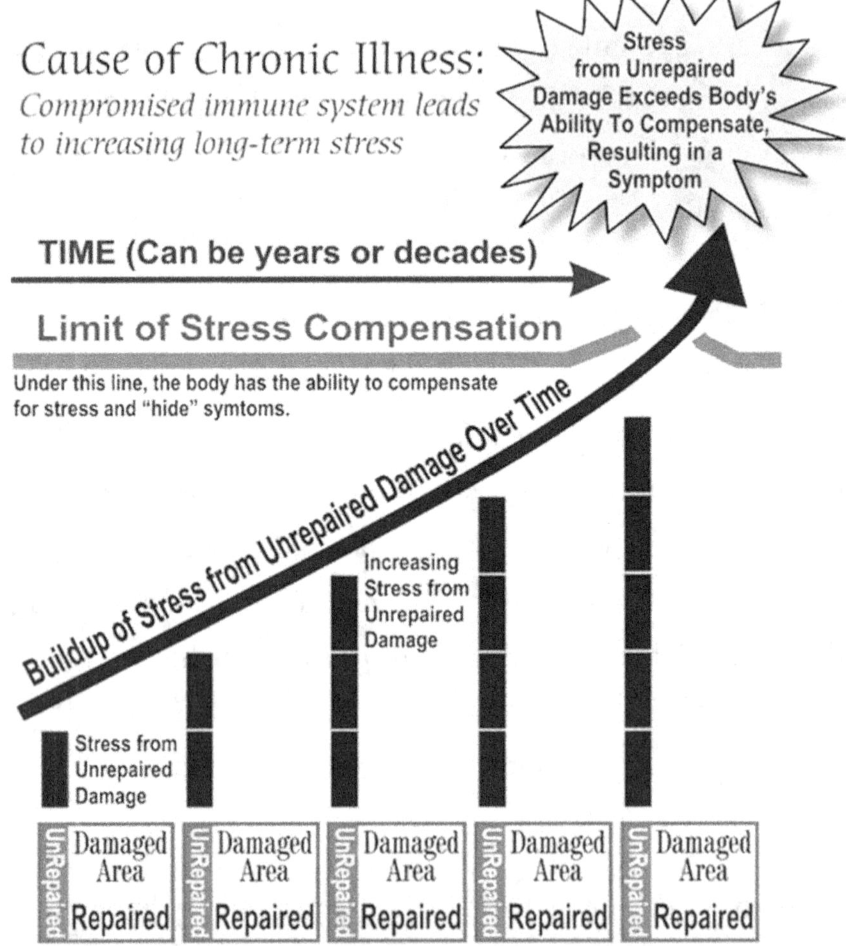

Compromised immune and digestive systems prevent body from completely healing normally occurring damage.

> **Over time, the body continues to develop unrepaired damage, creating an increase in permanent stress. This leads to additional chronic symptoms showing up, adding to the person's "permanent collection" of symptoms.**

Result: a long-term declining health trend.

This trend may be short- or long-term. I have had many patients who have told me that they feel their health has been declining their entire life. Others can track their decline to a stressful event, such as an injury or emotionally stressful period of their lives.

POSSIBLE SOLUTIONS

As the symptoms increase in frequency and intensity, you may reach a "Decision Point" where you realize something must be done about your health. Most patients tell me that fear of their health continuing to worsen is as important as the discomfort of the symptoms in reaching this point.

Health Outcomes Chart
The Future of Your Health

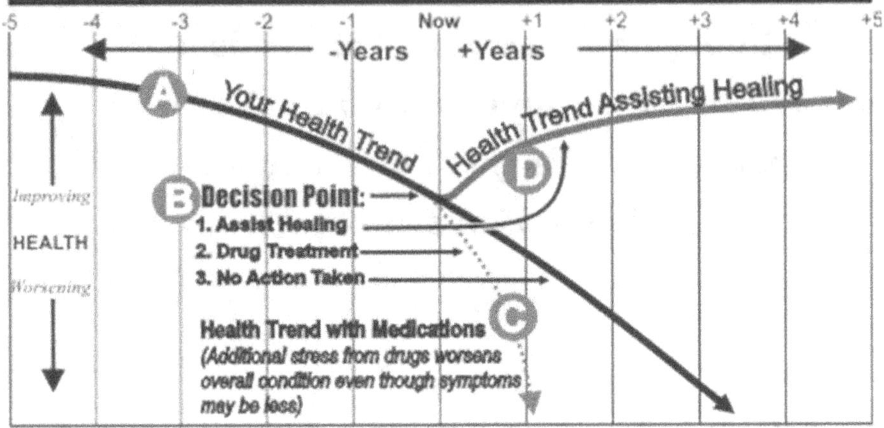

A **Your current health trend.** *If you have ongoing health problems, your long-term health trend may be worsening, like this graph.*

B **The Decision Point.** *When you realize that you are getting worse and that you must have a real, workable solution to recover your health.*

C **Your health trend on medications.** *You could go the medical route, the "tour of specialists." This may help to control symptoms, but the stress from the drugs may worsen your overall health more rapidly.*

D **Restoring your body's healing ability can completely change your health trend.** *Assisting your body's natural healing can be an effective method of changing your health trend from worsening to improving.*

The Four Possible Responses to a Chronic Health Problem

1. **Decide nothing can be done**, give up and live with their condition of declining health.

2. **Accept whatever medical help is available**. I sometimes call this the "Tour of Specialists." If you take *whatever* drugs and do *whatever* procedures are recommended medically, your symptoms might be

somewhat less, but the stress of the medical treatment and drugs will steepen the decline of your health. Often, I've had patients tell me that they tried all medical treatments without much success, gave up, and opted for #1 (live with it).

3. **Continue to live with the declining health condition**, but keep trying a long string of treatments and products that "might help." This approach can cause some symptoms to improve short-term, but the overall health trend usually stays the same—downward. The person may feel better by thinking that they are "doing something about" their health. Often people will justify their worsening health by blaming their age or genetics, or by observing how common their complaints are. None of this will help to recover health, quality of life or future health.

4. Another solution would be to **address the actual cause of the health decline: *the body's compromised immune systems.*** If this is successful, the body will rapidly transition from steadily worsening to beginning to improve. Bodies either get worse or get better, and if enough assistance is given to a body, it will stop worsening and begin to improve, typically over just a few weeks. If an effective program to assist the body to regain its ability to heal is

maintained over a long enough time, the body will continue to improve and will stabilize. At this point, a life-long program of supporting any permanent weakness can result in long-term stability and good health, with little attention on the body and maximum attention on life, all at a tiny fraction of the cost and pain of many conventional medical solutions.

> ***It should be evident that out of these choices, #4 would be the most productive and make the most sense. Yet, this is by far the least likely choice to be made.***

Here's why:

1. **These facts are not broadly known or publicized**, so few people discover this option.

2. **It requires a professional with specialized knowledge** and training. As this is not a well-known field, there are not a large number of practitioners trained and experienced to help you. Finding a qualified professional in a convenient location can be challenging.

3. **It requires a lot of personal responsibility** and willingness to change diets and lifestyles long-term. Another factor is that health insurance rarely covers any part of this type of health solution. Health insurance for the most part pays for drugs and surgery, but won't pay for a genuine solution to chronic health problems that will end the need for more treatment.

4. **Our current system of health care has created false but almost universally believed "facts" that act as traps,** preventing you from being able to see a way out of your chronic illness problems.

THE MOST COMMON TRAPS

Here are some of the traps that can prevent you from being able to see the truth about your own body and recovering your life and health.

THE "DIAGNOSIS" TRAP

I have heard thousands of patients voice some version of, *"If I knew what was causing my problem, I might be able to figure out how to get well."*

This is a very true statement. However, in our current health care system, asking the question, "What is wrong with me?" can spring a trap that can prevent you from ever recovering—*The Diagnosis Trap.*

This trap works by giving your health problem a name, and then substituting the name as the cause of the problem. For example, a doctor diagnoses you with "diabetes" and you now know you are a "diabetic." What is the cause of you being a diabetic? It's because you have diabetes! This circular thinking has zip to do with the actual cause of diabetes, and leads only to long-term drug treatment (which is what 85.3% of diabetics wind up with (CDC)).[6]

NOTE: *To clarify, Type II Diabetes is usually a reversible condition, a fact well known in traditional medicine as well as with alternative practitioners. The common practice of railroading a person with a diagnosis of diabetes onto a drug treatment program without even mentioning the option of lifestyle changes to reverse the condition entirely is a good example of the* **Diagnosis Trap** *in action.*

People may spend a great deal of time going from doctor to doctor trying to get a diagnosis in the mistaken belief that this will identify the treatment needed to get well. With chronic conditions, this rarely turns out to be the case. You may indeed get a diagnosis and a treatment for that diagnosis, but this is very, very unlikely to result in a resolution of your chronic health problem.

A diagnosis is a name for a specific symptom or group of symptoms. It generally has little or nothing to do with what is preventing the body from healing. Treatments for chronic diseases are usually drugs or surgeries, with the goal of *managing the symptoms or suppressing them*, not helping the body to heal.

Ask your doctor this question: "Doctor, what really CAUSES (name of disease)?" You'll usually get the answers of "your age," "your genetics" or "we don't really know." Essentially, your doctor is telling you the solution to your problem is to get younger or change your parents.

> ***Chronic health conditions are caused by specific stresses that your body lacks the resources to address and correct, not names of diseases.***

THE "FIX ME" TRAP

If you are caught in this trap, you've succumbed to the idea that there must be a "fix" for your problem, if only you could locate it! The truth is, there is no "fix" to a chronic health condition, if "fix" is defined as "quick and someone else does if for me."

The belief that there is a "fix" to a long-term health problem is partly rooted in drug company marketing. All drug ads push the line that "If you have symptoms, you are sick and need treatment (drugs). If your symptoms lessen or go away with the drug, now you are healthy (even if you have to continue to take the drug)." Every drug ad shows happy people recovered from their problems because they are taking a drug. This is the thinking that allows a person to take a drug for high blood pressure every day for the rest of his life and believe that he doesn't have a health problem. This same person might believe that his high blood pressure condition went away as soon as he started the drug, and that now it's fixed! The truth is that the drug only suppresses the symptom, leaving the underlying condition to worsen and stressing the body with a toxic drug.

Chronic health conditions typically evolve over many years. You may have had health problems for a decade or more *before* you had symptoms. Your body is very, very good at compensating, working around problems and hiding symptoms. By the time it runs out of options and can't hide the stresses from you any longer, there is a *lot* of damage to repair, which will usually take it many years to accomplish. There's no "quick fix" available because the problem took years to develop and simply can't be fixed quickly.

There is no quick "fix," no drug or surgery that will make you "like it never happened." There is only healing, which takes time and discipline from *you*. The longer you believe in the "fix" fiction, the longer it will take you to get started on the process of healing (indeed, if you ever do). Meanwhile, your condition will likely continue to worsen.

> **Chronic health conditions take a long time to develop and a long time to heal. A rule of thumb on this would be at least three months of healing for every year you have been aware of your problem.**

THE "AGREEMENT" TRAP

This may be the most common Trap to be caught in and the most difficult to overcome. This trap can be stated simply in three steps:

1. There is no medical (drug or surgery) solution to your chronic health problem.

2. The general public, the health care system, and likely your doctor and most of your family and friends, believe

that *only* medical care is legitimate. Everything else is useless at best, and a quackery and a scam at worst.

3. Therefore, if you feel you must have agreement from your doctor, family and friends as to how you approach your health problem, you may be stuck in the Agreement Trap. *All you can get agreement with are things that will not work.*

The easiest way out of this trap is to understand *why* your friends and family agree with medical treatment and disagree with anything else:

- Most people certainly don't want to leave the comfort of believing that the medical system can take care of them if they get sick. To discover they're on their own would be very scary.

- Your friends see all those people in the TV drug ads and how much happier they are since they tried that new drug. This reinforces the "drugs are the only legitimate treatment" idea. Multiply this by about 2.4 billion dollars spent annually just on direct-to-consumer television advertising on pharmaceuticals.[7]

- Doctors are seen in our society as larger-than-life, considered by most to be "the Health EXPERTS." Health care is a huge business—giant buildings, complex technical equipment, billions of dollars, difficult to pronounce words and complicated names of diseases. Then there are all those prestigious medical schools that are hard to get into and charge hundreds of thousands in tuition. Research is done by PhDs in big, expensive labs and written up in prestigious journals that are respected worldwide. You see all this impressive infrastructure; you see people's lives being saved by all the high-level technology.

> **It's hard to imagine that there is a hole in medicine the size of: "Half the population is sick and the experts have no answers."**

The difficult-to-face truth is that despite the prestige, money, training, degrees and respect, *medicine has no real solution for your chronic health problem.*

Therefore, to be successful in recovering your health you're going to have to just let other people have their opinions, know what you know, keep your own counsel and find a non-medical solution to your health problems.

Finding other people to talk to who really understand the problems you are dealing with and agree with the methods you have chosen to recover is a key part of getting your health back. Standing on your own against the agreement of what can seem like the entire society can be daunting. The more support you have, the more likely you will recover your health.

THE "COMPLACENCY" TRAP

Complacency: *a feeling of quiet pleasure or security, often while unaware of some potential danger or defect.*

This is the most common health trap you can fall in to.

Your body is designed to take care of itself with minimum attention from you. If it develops a problem, it will hide that problem as long as possible, until the stress becomes overwhelming. This makes it easy to imagine that your health is good, when "under the covers" your body is hanging on by a thread.

In this trap, you are lulled into thinking that your health is fine, and you can ignore the health carnage going on all around you using the "it won't happen to me, hey—I feel fine right now!" argument.

In our society, we mainly see health in three phases:

1. **Bad**. "I am/will shortly get treatment to take care of my symptoms."

2. **Needs Improvement**. "I am/should eat better and exercise to improve my health."

3. **Good**. "Health? I'm doing great!"

When your health is good, it's easy to believe it will always be this way and simply ignore it.

If you'll examine any and every part of this world, you'll find that everything either improves or gets worse. Nothing stays the same very long. Even rocks and mountains erode and deteriorate.

If you don't take some action to keep your health improving, even if you don't have symptoms, it will eventually deteriorate.

This is even more true if you've recovered from a previous condition of poor health or a major health problem. In this case, not continuously working to improve your health is guaranteed to result in a relapse into poor health.

To maintain good health, you must take actions to keep it continuously improving.

UNDERSTANDING HOW BODIES HEAL

How your body can become stuck and unable to heal, and how it's possible to assist it back to normal recovery and health.

Your body is designed to heal itself. If you are experiencing ongoing symptoms that aren't improving, you can be sure that your body is trying its best to heal but has become *stuck* in the healing process.

Getting a stuck body back to healing relies on the body itself to do the repairs. **Your role in this is to be an effective assistant**, helping the body by giving it what it needs to start healing again.

- The first step: Arrange for accurate testing to find out where your body is stuck and what it needs to start healing again.

- Second step: As an assistant you would hand over to your body the needed material that was found in the testing so the body can move itself past the stuck point and get on with the healing process.

This is a repetitive action. Remember all those work-arounds from when your body couldn't heal all the way? Each of these can stick the body again and stop further healing progress. When you help the body remove a barrier, it will continue to heal—until it hits the next barrier it can't get past. You'd then need to test and find out where this new stuck point is and what's needed this time to unstick it to get your body resuming its healing progress.

Each time your body moves past a previously stuck area, it's healthier and has more energy and a greater ability to heal. You could say that it moves farther each time toward a condition of stable good health, until finally you don't have to help it anymore. Your body would now be back to being able to heal, allowing it to repair old damage as well as handle any new stresses that happen from the normal process of living life.

OK... But I don't know how to do any of this...

Yes, you are going to need some professional help.

> **Recovering from a serious chronic health condition based on trial-and-error, advice from friends, self-help books and Dr. Google is long, expensive and ultimately likely to fail.**

Out of the four actions you could take having reached a Decision Point on your health, this is #3: *"Continue to live with the declining health condition, but keep trying a long string of treatments and products that "might help."*

Often, a patient will complain to me, *"I keep reading about people who get better using all kinds of self-treatment and products they buy at the health food store and on the internet, or by changing their diets, like going gluten- and dairy-free. But this hasn't ever worked for me."*

People get results from various solutions because health problems come in different levels of severity.

In a simple case, a specific area of stress may exceed the body's ability to compensate and create a symptom, but few other areas of the body are particularly stressed. In this case, the body can sort itself out over time and recover to a lower-stress condition without chronic symptoms. Supplements or treatments that reduce stress *anywhere in the body* can help to speed this process, as the body is a closed system and less stress in one area can translate into more resources to heal another area.

For example: "Jane" has a minor but symptomatic thyroid stress and is suffering from mental sluggishness and anxiety, constipation, dry skin and menstrual problems. Jane takes some vitamins and minerals, removes gluten from her diet and starts exercising. These actions may reduce physical stress, as well as lessening her mental stress because she feels that by living a healthier lifestyle she is doing something about her problem. Her body might use the newly freed-up resources from her stress-reducing actions to compensate for the thyroid problem—and her symptoms could improve. Jane writes on her blog how her actions "are the solution to healing thyroid symptoms." She's making the error of thinking that what worked for her will work for anyone.

"Ann" reads this blog and feels hope, as she has similar symptoms. However, Ann has a serious thyroid problem caused by an autoimmune condition (where the body's immune system is attacking healthy tissue; in this case, it's ripping up her thyroid), compounded by adrenal failure and long-term digestive problems. Ann does all the things that Jane recommends, but sees no improvement at all.

Ann may spend years trying other methods, supplements, diets and treatments with no stable or meaningful improvement.

What's missing in her case is:

- Accurate testing and a correct assessment of exactly why her body can't heal and identifying the stresses that are creating this situation.

- An organized system of using this testing information to effectively help her body to heal.

If you are frustrated because none of the "cures" you've read about that have worked for others have worked for you, your case is likely more severe and may not recover without specific testing and treatment from a competent professional.

Many of my patients have come to me after years of trying different medical and non-medical solutions, none of which did anything beyond short-term symptom relief.

EVECTICS℠, AN ENTIRELY NEW APPROACH TO HEALTH CARE

> *I have developed a health improvement technique that adapts to every aspect of the individual case. This completely customized approach is a radical departure from traditional and alternative medicine techniques.*

This section of the book outlines the **Evectics℠** system of healing and how it works. If you have become frustrated by health problems that haven't resolved, you may take hope from this organized and precise system based on testing and physiology instead of opinion or the ridged dogma of pharmaceutical-based medicine.

In the 1800s, the word "evectics" (e VEK tics) meant, "The branch of medical science which teaches the method of acquiring a good habit of body."* In other words, evectics meant "the method of obtaining health." The word went out of use in the early 1900s, as medicine became more about relief of symptoms and less about health. I have resurrected it as a name for my system of individualized health improvement therapy.

*"Good habit of body" means that the body is well-constructed and attractive. A definition of "habit" is "bodily appearance or makeup."

Evectics^SM Consists of Four Main Parts:

- Clinical Nutrition (with many variations)

- Specific, targeted diet improvements

- Two major acupressure techniques (with many variations)

- Lab testing (blood, saliva, urine, dried urine, stool, etc.)

THE ROLE OF NUTRITION IN HEALING

"Eat healthy to be healthy." "You are what you eat." You've heard these clichés. Most people I talk to are at least aware that food has something to do with their health, but I don't think

I've ever come across the individual who could state exactly why this is.

A good example of this is a question I often use in public talks. I'll ask the group, "Can anyone define the word *food*?" Someone will say, "What you eat,"——easily wrong, as you can certainly eat things that aren't food. Someone else will volunteer, "Stuff you eat that gives you energy." While this is true, it's far from a complete definition, kind of like defining "book" as "source of entertainment." Not the whole story by any means. This usually continues for a while until the group comes to the realization that they can't really come up with a good definition for "food." Then I'll give them the actual definition, what food really is: *The living, fresh or preserved tissue of plants and animals.*

This definition is always highly unsatisfying to the group; they can't understand why this would be true. So I give them a quick series of facts to sort it out:

Your body is made of cells.

The average cell in your body only lives for about three months. Look at your face in the mirror; it's all less than three months old!

During the time it takes you to read this sentence, your body has flushed out and rebuilt 5 million cells (that's an average rate of 96 million cells per minute).

New cells to replace the dead ones are assembled by your body from component parts. These component parts are made from sunlight and soil, but you don't have any leaves or roots, and therefore, *can't make the parts for your own cells.*

The component parts your body must have to make new cells come from eating and digesting the tissue from plants and animals that do have the materials necessary to make cells.

Your entire body is being constantly rebuilt from the food you eat—if you define "food" *as "living, fresh or preserved tissue of plants and animals."*

So to quote the cliché, you really are "what you eat!"

> **Because nutrition is the raw material your body is made of, any successful technique to help the body to heal itself from chronic problems must rely in part or in whole on nutrition.**

Let's chart out the process of assisting your body to recover its health:

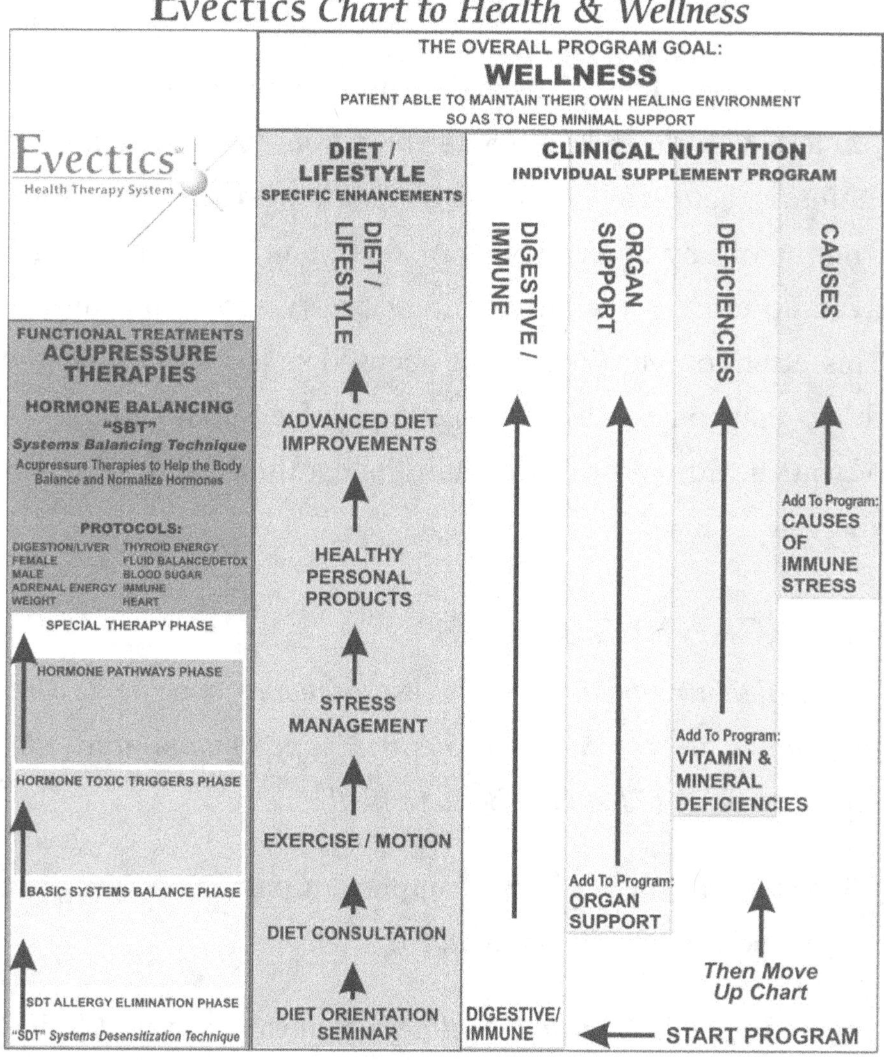

This Chart shows how bodies heal. Most of our patients start at or near the bottom of the chart (at "Start Program" on the

Chart). Our goal is to help them to help their body to heal its way up to the top of the chart.

The final goal for your health:

To have your body healthy and continuing to improve, and for you to have enough knowledge about your body to be able to *maintain your own improving health* with very little help from us or any other doctor. At this point, you should have freed up most of the attention and worry about your health. This attention can instead be focused on your life and the things that you care about, because you feel you are in control of your health and can maintain its continued improvement yourself.

CLINICAL NUTRITION*

**Clinical Nutrition is the process of using specific testing techniques to recommend dietary supplements and diet improvements to help the body to heal.*

Clinical Nutrition is the most important part of any program to get a body back to healing itself.

On the *Chart to Health & Wellness*, you can see that Clinical Nutrition consists of four separate areas or *levels* of healing:

Digestive / Immune: Your digestive system is 70% of your immune system and makes up most of your body's ability to repair and maintain itself. When this area becomes compromised, your body can't heal completely, which leads to chronic health conditions. The first action to assist your body to heal is to help the digestive and immune systems begin to function more efficiently.

Organ Support: If you have chronic health problems, your body almost certainly has many organs that are malfunctioning but can't be repaired (which is why you don't recover your health). The most basic reason for this is that your digestive and immune systems are insufficient. Once these systems begin to come back on line, your body will use its new healing resources to begin to repair the organ systems.

Deficiencies: Once your organ systems are starting to function better, your body can start to improve any deficiencies it has developed. Most vitamin and mineral deficiencies are caused by damage to organ systems and won't improve until those organs and glands are repaired. Damaged organs can't process and absorb the nutrients, leading to deficiencies. For example, if you are deficient in calcium, it will do you no good to take any amount of calcium supplements if your thyroid and parathyroid glands can't convert calcium carbonate into blood calcium.

Causes: Somewhere in your history, your body developed a stress that it could not heal or compensate for. This stress continued to cause damage to your body over time, leading eventually to the chronic state you find yourself in now. Once you have healed "up the Chart" to this level, your body will have the resources and energy to heal or compensate in this area to some degree. When this stress has been reduced, it's possible for your health to be much more stable and continue to improve.

How Your Body Rebuilds Itself

As you learned in grammar school, your body is made of cells. This means the parts of your body are made of cells as well. *The overall health of your cells creates the overall health of your body.*

For example, if your stomach isn't functioning correctly, you might experience cramping, reflux, gas and bloating. The reason for the poor function of your stomach is that it is made up of *too many cells that are damaged or unhealthy.*

If your body was to heal or repair your stomach, it wouldn't use tiny screwdrivers to fix it; instead, it would *remodel* the stomach. It would replace enough of the damaged and unhealthy cells with healthier versions of those cells until the organ could function at a normal level. You've seen this remodeling in action when you've scraped your elbow: your body sloughs off the damaged tissue and "remodels" the damaged area into a new, pink, healthy elbow. This is what happens internally as well.

A Huge Clue

Here's a huge clue as to why your body hasn't been able to heal: *The average lifespan of a cell in your body is only about three months.* Using the previous example, this means that your body has completely rebuilt your stomach many times—but something is preventing it from being restored to full function. The evidence is that your body has been unable to rebuild your stomach any healthier than its current state. Your body knows how to rebuild itself, but it's failing to do the job properly. This shows that there is a *supply problem*: the materials your body needs to rebuild the stomach cells just aren't available or can't be used correctly.

What are cells made of, anyway? What is it that your body needs to rebuild these cells that it can't get?

Cells are made of *component parts* that the body assembles into finished cells. These parts come mainly from sunlight and soil, but since you don't have any leaves or roots, your body can't make the component parts needed to make its own cells. To get the components needed you must eat the cellular material from other lifeforms that have leaves and roots. Then your digestive system must separate out these com-ponents and put them into your bloodstream, so your body can make new cells.

The component parts that make up your body are _nutrition_.

Now you can more fully understand the process I was discussing earlier, where we find the stuck point in the healing process and then assist the body to move past that point. *The only way to move the body past a stuck point is to supply the specific nutrition required to rebuild that area.* If you were fixing a car, you wouldn't argue that you'd replace the parts till it worked correctly. The same is true with your body—it's just that body parts are *nutrition.*

There are specific reasons why your body might not be able to get the parts it needs:

- Possibly you aren't eating them or the food supply itself is deficient.

- Possibly your digestive system isn't working well enough to break down the food, remove the cellular components and supply them into the bloodstream.

- Possibly there are stresses or malfunctions in your body that are using up so much of a nutrient that the body just can't get enough.

Clinical Nutrition is the process of testing the body to find:

- Where it's stuck

- Exactly what nutrients are required to assist the body past the stuck point

These nutrients must then be made available in the form of supplements and improved diet.

Once this has been done, the body will be able to move past the stuck point, and as I mentioned before, it will improve but will shortly get stuck again on the next unresolved area of stress.

Because of this, Clinical Nutrition is a *repetitive process*, testing and supplementing, then retesting and adjusting the supplements. This is done until the body gets healthy enough not to require ongoing assistance in healing.

Although Clinical Nutrition is the most important part of any healing program, there's more to recovering the health of a patient with severe chronic health problems than just giving them the right supplements. *There are other barriers that can prevent Clinical Nutrition itself from working to help heal the body.*

Clinical Nutrition Process

CONTINUOUSLY IMPROVING, STABLE HEALTH (End of Process)

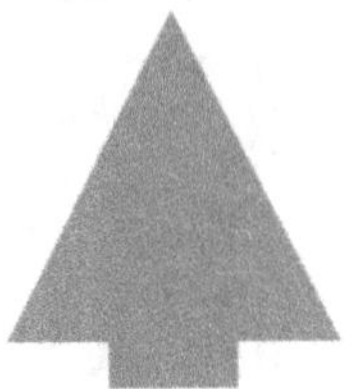

Body Has Regained the Ability to Heal Itself, Requires only Support Supplements for Areas of Permanent Damage

Un-Repaired Body Damage

Body Sticks Again, But Continues to Improve

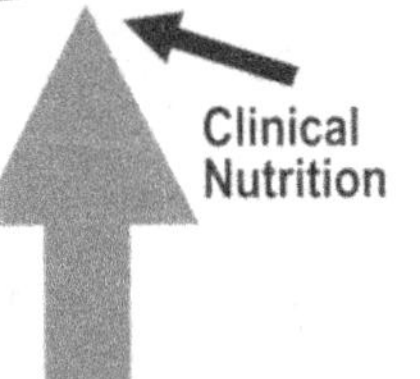

These Cycles May Continue For Months or Years until the Body can Heal Without Assistance

Un-Repaired Body Damage

Body Sticks Again, But Continues to Improve

Clinical Nutrition is Adjusted to Assist with This Different Damage

Un-Repaired Body Damage

Body Sticks Again, But is in Better Condition Now

Clinical Nutrition is Adjusted to Assist with This Different Damage

Un-Repaired Body Damage

Body is Stuck, Unable to Heal Damaged Area

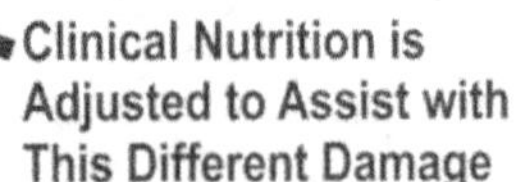

Clinical Nutrition "Assist" of Supplements and Improved Diet Allows Body to Move Through Barrier

CHRONIC ILLNESS (Start of Process)

DIET AND LIFESTYLE

Diet: Oxford dictionary—the origin of the word "diet" is Greek—diaita—which means "a way of life."

> **I often tell people that they are trying to climb up the *Chart to Health & Wellness* as if it was a ladder, but they're struggling with their climb because of wearing a concrete backpack from their diet.**

Great improvements have been made in the past decades in helping the public to understand that food is related to health. Counter to this improvement has been the government and private sector using false information about "how to eat healthy" to further their own agendas. We've been falsely informed that eggs are unhealthy, that fat is bad, that low-fat and low-cholesterol foods are healthy and that bread, pasta and other refined carbohydrates are the basis of any healthy diet (all these are false). Toxic food additives to preserve and improve flavor, odor and appearance are fully accepted and generally ignored as the health threat that they really are.

As a direct result of this misinformation, there is an epidemic of chronic health conditions such as heart disease, cancer, obesity, diabetes and the myriad health conditions related to these.

THE SECRET TO SUCCESSFUL LONG-TERM DIET IMPROVEMENT

In 20+ years of experience, I've learned that helping my patients to eat a diet that will allow their bodies to heal with Clinical Nutrition is often the most difficult part of their entire treatment program.

Telling people what to eat is never a workable solution.

Everyone has different tastes, needs and food logistics, and these often change. However, *unless dietary stress is reduced, healing won't occur.* Also, a healthy diet that supports the weak areas in a patient's body is the single most important factor in long-term stable health.

It's critically necessary that patients eat in a way that doesn't prevent their bodies from healing, but how can people succeed in changing their behavior long-term?

For years I struggled with this problem while my patients struggled with their diets.

Then, I had a bright idea. I noticed that almost everyone obeys some dietary guidelines based on an *understanding of commonly-known facts about how food affects the body's health.*

For example, I'll bet you don't drink dirty water. Even if you're thirsty and the only water available is dirty, you still don't drink it. You understand that bacteria and toxins in dirty water can make you sick, and based on this understanding you avoid drinking it. You can probably think of several other examples of your diet being influenced by an understanding of how your body is affected by food.

So instead of telling my patients what to eat, I educate them about *how the food they eat affects their body's ability to heal.* This is:

- **Interesting**: Really, it's very cool information. It's not difficult to understand and doesn't rely on a background of education in science or biology.

- **You only make the most important changes**. There are probably thousands of legitimate dietary improvements that might work. But I have learned that people can only make limited changes in their life, so they should spend their "change" wisely! My experience is that focusing on a half-dozen improve-ments is usually all that's needed.

- **It WORKS!** When you modify your diet based on this information, your Clinical Nutrition program really kicks in, and you see results. The better you eat, the faster you heal. Also, when you slip up, you notice that you feel worse. It doesn't take long to realize that what I've taught you is 1) True, and 2) Effective.

- **YOU decide what to eat**: This is the whole idea—that based on having this information you can make your own food choices in many different circum-stances. Because you're in control and educated, you understand why you are making these choices. Because it works and you feel better, you won't stop eating this way. The patients I talk to from a decade ago still report they are eating the same way and loving it.

The real solution to eating well so you don't stress your body and prevent healing is to **work out how you can enjoy your new diet more than how you used to eat**. If you accomplish this, you will never go back to eating poorly.

Remember: the origin of the word "diet" is Greek—diaita—which means "a way of life."

HOW REDUCING FUNCTIONAL STRESS SPEEDS HEALING

Beyond the stress from a poor diet, the second barrier to healing with a Clinical Nutrition program is *functional stress.*

Function in the body is how it operates. Digesting food, moving muscles, controlling metabolism are all body *functions.* All functions operate under the control of the two internal body communication systems:

- The nervous system

- The hormone system

For example, your muscles move because an electrical signal passed through the nervous system instructing them to do so. Digestive processes are controlled by both the chemical hormone system and the electrical nervous system.

When these communication systems break down or become inefficient, your body develops a *functional stress.* Sex hormone problems, thyroid problems, blood sugar problems (such as diabetes), blood pressure problems, difficulty sleeping, digestive issues, etc. all are mainly functional problems created by a breakdown of the body's communication systems.

*In every case with which I have experience, chronic health conditions involve both **structural** problems (damaged or* *unhealthy cells) and **functional** problems from the hormone and/or nervous systems.*

The main sources of interference in the hormone and nervous systems are:

- Toxins (including chemicals, metals, fungus, bacteria, virus, etc.)

- Sensitivities and allergies.

Toxins tend to affect mainly the hormone system while sensitivities mainly stress the nervous system.

When you begin to help your body to heal nutritionally, you add stress to any damaged functional systems. It's like having bald tires on your car. If you are going slowly, there's no issue. But if you fix your engine and start getting up to highway speeds, the stress on the tires increases and they may blow out.

A Clinical Nutrition program by itself without any help for functional stresses may hang up at some point, due to the increase in demand for function as the body heals and begins to increase its operations. In most cases, the speed of body healing can be increased by reducing functional stress.

Delivering specific functional treatments, along with a Clinical Nutrition treatment program, prevents the healing process from hanging up and stopping and can greatly speed up healing by removing functional barriers.

Functional therapies can be used on an as-needed basis to unstick a Clinical Nutrition program and speed it up. These therapies aren't for symptom relief and they won't get you well by themselves. They are done to keep your progress going up the *Chart to Health & Wellness.* You can see that if you continue to move up the Chart and become healthy enough that eventually symptom relief efforts aren't going to be needed, anyway.

Below, see the complete *Chart to Health & Wellness,* including functional therapies. We have found that the best and most rapid results with patients are achieved with:

- Clinical Nutrition

- Diet Improvements

- Functional Therapies

All three delivered at the same time.

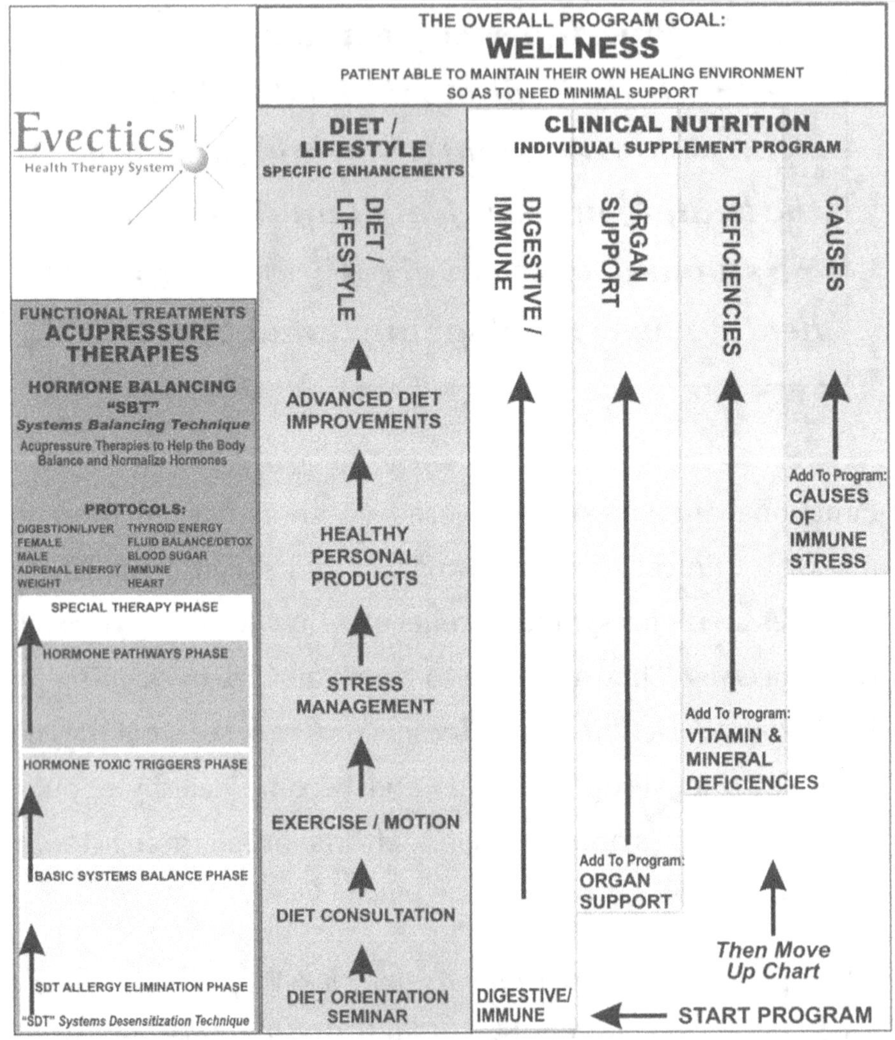

FUNCTIONAL TREATMENTS, the final column on the chart:

Evectics[SM] functional treatments are **acupressure therapies**. *Acupressure* is acupuncture technology using low-powered laser and light finger pressure instead of needles.

Acupuncture is a technique of directing the attention of the body to specific areas, organs and systems. *Acupressure* does this as well. By directing the body to "look at" allergies and areas of toxic stress causing hormone imbalances, we can help the body to correct its own stress.

There are two main acupressure functional techniques, each with many variations:

Systems Desensitization Technique ("SDT") helps the body to resolve misidentification problems, such as allergies. For example, SDT helps the body to stop misidentifying an allergic food as stressful, and to see it instead as it is—a harmless and beneficial food. This can reduce or eliminate any reactions and reduce stress to assist in the healing process. SDT can also help the body to reduce excessive stress caused by overreactions to pathogens like bacteria or viruses, or to toxins like heavy metals or chemicals.

Systems Balancing Technique ("SBT") helps the body to resolve hormone stress caused by imbalances, toxins and chemical confusions. SBT has specific protocols for many areas of stress, such as female sex hormones, heart, digestive, blood sugar, adrenals, thyroid and many more. A very useful application of SBT is *cravings therapies*, used to help reduce sugar, carbohydrate and junk food cravings. We use these therapies to make it much easier for patients to eat in a way that reduces stress and promotes healing.

We use all three columns on the chart simultaneously with patients. A patient will be tested (ongoing) for the correct supplements, helped to eat a diet that won't stop the healing process and we will do appropriate functional acupressure therapies.

PUTTING IT ALL TOGETHER

Routinely helping patients with long-term chronic health conditions to accomplish a recovery for themselves is done by using:

- Clinical Nutrition

- Dietary Improvements

- Functional Therapies

But, this is a bit like saying a car is made of wheels, a body and an engine. It takes a lot of exact engineering and manufacturing expertise to make a car, far beyond these basics.

Every patient is different and requires a unique therapy program. As the patient's body heals, the need for correct assistance to maintain healing changes as well. We address these needs by creating a custom program based on a patient's health history, nervous system testing, lab testing and the health goals of that patient. Then, as the patient heals and their body changes, we adjust their program to **keep helping the body to heal** at maximum speed.

Programming in an **Evectics**[SM] therapy program is done on different levels:

- **Overall programming** to keep the program on long-term goals and consistent with the major stresses present in the patient's body.

- **Mid-range programming** to help the body address the current stresses that are being worked through right now.

- **Visit programming** to deal with immediate needs such as dietary stress, short-term toxic stress (such as the fast food chemicals the patient unfortunately ate yesterday), and acute factors.

THE CARE FACTOR

> **I can state categorically that a *patient will not recover unless that person is in very good communication with their practitioner*.**

Poor communication means the patient may misunderstand or not understand instructions, do the wrong things or fail to do the right things needed to heal.

There's only one way to be in good communication with a patient: *You must really care about them and like them!* This results in the patient caring and liking the practitioner as well. How well do you communicate with someone you don't like? Not so good, correct?

Good communication is a direct result of liking and caring.

A patient may have difficulty doing some part of their program and may need help. The best help a practitioner can give is to be on their patient's team! If the patient feels they have a responsibility to get well and to do their program very well, that their practitioner cares about them and will be excited for their success, this can overcome a lot of difficulty the patient may be experiencing in making the changes in their life that are needed to heal.

Our sad medical system suffers from short visits and overworked doctors who can come off as not caring. They often aren't in good communication with their patients, a fact that leads to many devastating medical errors.

HOW EVECTICS^{SM} DIFFERS FROM TRADITIONAL MEDICINE

To help you understand this new technology, this chapter is a comparison between how **Evectics^{SM}** handles chronic health problems compared to traditional medicine.

EVECTICS^{SM}: TESTING, UNDERSTANDING, AND THEN THERAPY

With **Evectics^{SM}**, the first action with a patient is to *test* the patient. Decades of experience with difficult cases has taught me that anything can happen in a case and that I must test thoroughly before any therapy is even planned.

Rather than test just the areas associated with your complaint, I test the body overall to determine *why your body cannot heal.* This is fundamentally different from the medical approach, which is based on symptoms (including symptoms that show up on labs. Your blood test values are *symptoms;* they are not causing the health problems that created them).

Once I know which areas of your body are stressed and the cause of that stress, your entire case history, current and past symptoms and other factors that can affect healing, I'm ready to choose the specific tools required in your case and create a customized program.

This approach is a dramatic departure from other medical and alternative approaches to diagnosis and treatment.

EVECTICS℠ USES INDIVIDUALIZED THERAPY

Your body needs the treatment it needs, even if your doctor only knows how to do something else.

"If you only have a hammer, you tend to see every problem as a nail." — Abraham Maslow

It is completely amazing to me that this isn't obvious to everyone.

If you go to a:

- **Medical doctor**, you will likely leave with a prescription for a drug.

- **Chiropractor**, you will almost certainly receive a chiropractic adjustment.

- **Nutritionist**, you will probably get a recommendation for supplements and vitamins.

- **Acupuncturist**, you'll get an acupuncture treatment.

You will receive a treatment based on what the doctor you happen to go to knows how to do, not based on what your body may need to heal. In many cases, patients are "going to a plumber for an electrical problem" but don't realize this, because the plumber imagines he can fix your wiring.

Bodies with complex problems often need many different types of treatment. This explains one reason that your chronic problem may change somewhat under conventional or alternative treatment but never resolves. Your treatment with a doctor may or may not be incorrect, but if you are under only one type of treatment when your body needs several, you will get incomplete results at best.

THE EVECTICS^{SM} TOOLKIT

Following is a list of some of the **Evectics**^{SM} tools. This is not a complete list, but it will give you an idea of some of the main tools I use:

- **Clinical Nutrition**: exact dietary supplements based on ongoing testing. There are four major divisions of this technique: Whole Food, Drainage, Homeopathy and Herbology.

- **SDT**— *Systems Desensitization Technique*: An acupressure technique (no needles, we use cold laser to stimulate the acupuncture points) to help the body recover from allergies, sensitivities, immune and inflammation issues and gut and digestive stress.

- **SBT**— *Systems Balancing Technique*: An acupressure technique (nine specific protocols) to help the body recover from hormone imbalances caused by toxins in the food and environment.

- **Diet/Lifestyle**: My program is focused on improving immune response, not "eating healthy." This approach can result in rapid improvement of a patient's problems as well as long-term health benefits without having someone else telling you what to eat.

- **Cravings Solutions**: Therapies to put *you* back in control of what you eat.

- **Heart Rate Variability** (HRV): Computerized testing of the autonomic nervous system (the private network that the body uses to run itself—digesting food, growing hair, healing, etc.) to identify and resolve nervous system problems that can prevent or slow the healing process.

- **Functional Lab Testing**: Most people are very familiar with *diagnostic testing*, which are the labs they get from their medical doctor. These labs show symptoms (high cholesterol, for example) that can be suppressed with a drug. A different approach to lab testing are *functional labs*, which include tests of blood, saliva, hair, urine and stool that are designed to give the doctor information related to how the body is functioning. This information, when used with other forms of testing and observing how the body responds to various therapies, can provide objective information on what tools the doctor should use and what approach the body will respond to and work with. Functional labs show objective improvement as the patient improves their lab values from the original baseline.

An **Evectics**[SM] practitioner has a full set of tools, not just one treatment method, and can use accurate testing and case programming to know exactly which tools to use, in what combination and in what order. This is a very important key to resolving chronic health problems.

EVECTICS^{SM} USES TESTING, NOT OPINION

The Medical Opinion

"One accurate measurement is worth a thousand expert opinions" — Admiral Grace Hopper

When a medical doctor is treating chronic health conditions, he or she often relies largely on their opinion of what is wrong and what treatment needs to be done. This is so true that it's normal to go get a "second opinion" to see if you can get more than one doctor to agree on your treatment.

My view is that measurement and testing should replace opinion. An opinion is really a guess.

Correct, effective Case Programming based on accurate testing is crucial. Using accurate testing to determine what therapies the body needs and in what order they are required is called "Case Programming." A well-done Case Program correctly interprets the testing and labs and does not rely on "the doctor's experience" or "opinion." The reason we do accurate testing is to develop a correct Case Program. The Case Program is a step-by-step written guide to resolving the patient's case.

Evectics[SM] practitioners are specifically trained in case programming and use exact testing and not guesswork. **Practitioners operate with the help of a highly trained Case Director** who checks programs, patient progress (quality control) and consults with practitioners. Patient progress is surveyed and measured at every visit, analyzed and graphed to find any slowdowns or inefficiencies and resolve them.

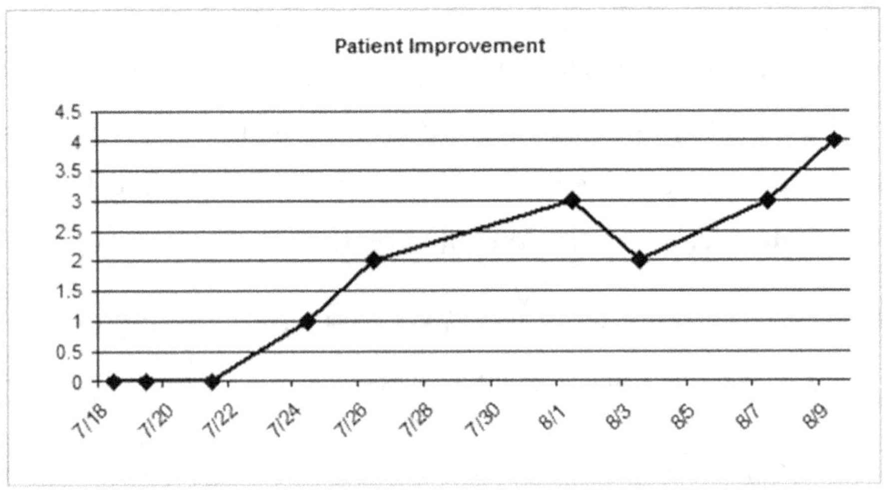

Evectics[SM] Patient Improvement Graph

WHEN ARE YOU "DONE" WITH A TREATMENT PROGRAM?

A question I often ask of doctors (both medical and alternative) is, "When do you know that your patient is DONE with their treatment program?" Here are a few answers I get regularly:

- "When they feel better and don't want to come in anymore."

- "When I have completed the standard treatment protocol." (Often regardless of outcome.)

- "When their insurance (or money) runs out."

- "If they don't respond well to my treatment, I refer them to a specialist."

None of these answers has much to do with regaining a stable **and improving** state of health.

Three Goals of an Evectics^{SM} treatment program

Here are three goals for a sensible treatment program that has as its aim the restoration of health rather than control of symptoms:

1. That the patient's body is no longer a problem in their life.

2. That the patient is not worried or anxious over what could happen to their health in the future.

3. That the patient feels confident in their knowledge and ability to live a lifestyle where they can maintain their own health **and improve it** from now on.

With these goals achieved to the satisfaction of the patient, they can be successfully graduated from a treatment program and monitored occasionally a few times a year on a wellness program to support any weak areas and catch and head off any developing health issues.

An **Evectics**ᔆᴹ program is complete when the patient is satisfied with the results and tests show the improvements are stable and should continue.

And it works!

During two decades of research and testing, I have helped patient's bodies to heal almost every type of health problem.

See AlternativeHealthAtlanta.com/testimonials (http://alternativehealthatlanta.com/testimonials/) for 800+ testimonials on dozens of different health problems.

What You Can Do Next:

I have developed an "**Evectics^{SM} Evaluation**," which is a very efficient **method of analysis** to determine:

1. What is preventing your body from healing

2. How it could be assisted back to health

3. What would be required to do this

Here is what is accomplished during this hour-long **analysis** session:

- Testing to determine if your ANS (Autonomic Nervous System) is malfunctioning in a way that will prevent your body from healing normally (and, if so, the cause and solution to this problem).

- Testing to determine your body's overall level of physiological function and remaining ability to adapt to stress.

- Testing to determine the areas (organs and systems) of your body that are stressed, which organ or system is the primary stress and the main cause of that stress?

- A comprehensive, in-depth consultation on your health history and current symptoms.

Once testing is complete, your practitioner and the Case Director will review all your information to write a Case Program specifically for you. This program will sequentially address the stresses preventing your body from healing based on your test results, using whatever techniques, products and lab tests are indicated.

NEXT:

You will make a second appointment to come back, once your Case Program has been completed. At this appointment, you will receive an in-depth consultation on both your test results and your Case Program. This consultation is educational and informational in nature and covers the physiology behind your body's inability to heal and the exact program steps that could resolve your case.

If we can accept your case, you will be given a written estimate of what an **Evectics**[SM] program at the clinic would require in time, scheduling and finance.

TO GET STARTED:

To schedule an Evectics[SM] Evaluation:

- *Call 770-612-1100 (new patient line) OR:*

- *Go to:* AlternativeHealthAtlanta.com/schedule-initial-visit/ *to request an appointment online*

- *Email us:* <u>HealthHelp@AlternativeHealthAtlanta.com</u>

If you would like some more information before you schedule an initial evaluation, you can take an online test on our website and submit it for a free phone consultation with a practitioner. Go to our homepage at

<u>https://AlternativeHealthAtlanta.com</u> and click the "Health Quiz" menu button to take the Life Quality Evaluation online test.

Have a Question? Call 770-612-1100 and ask for our new patient coordinator.

LAST THOUGHTS ON REGAINING HEALTH

Chronic health conditions can cause permanent damage to your body. Happily, bodies are designed with backup systems and an amazing ability to compensate for what can't be fully repaired—although the degree of healing available to any individual is certainly a case-by-case situation. The sooner you start the healing process, the less damage your body will have to repair.

Recovering your health from this kind of problem is almost never quick or easy. Should you decide to embark on a journey to regain your health, you should only do so with a lot of determination and a decidedly long-term view. Searching out a like-minded practitioner and clinic to support, guide and help you makes your chances of success improve dramatically.

I have a solution to assist your body to heal and recover. Seeing the results of this in the clinic every day is very exciting and rewarding. I invite you to contact us, get your questions answered, get tested, find out why your body isn't healing ... and then DO something effective about it! I would be very excited and happy to see you regain your health and look forward to hearing from you.

MY STORY: HOW EVECTICS^{SM} WAS DEVELOPED

From earliest childhood, I wanted to be a doctor—I declared this to my parents as soon as I could talk. I pursued school with a vengeance for top grades, so I could get into the best medical school. I continued this dedicated trajectory toward becoming a medical doctor right through my undergraduate degree. During the summer I spent studying for my MCAT test (Medical College Admission Test) to get into medical school, I took a part-time job at a local chiropractor's office. I had no idea what a chiropractor even was at the time, but his explanation shook me to my roots. "I help the body do what it was designed to do— heal *itself*. I remove interference from the nervous system, so the body can communicate and heal damage and disease."

The few months I spent working in the chiropractor's office changed my idea of what healthcare should be. Patients *wanted* to come to his clinic; they talked about their successes with each other as they worked to improve their own health. It was a happy, friendly, helpful place full of patients getting better because their own bodies were healing.

I compared this atmosphere to the medical offices that I had experience with—what a difference!

But it was the concept of the body healing itself with assistance from the doctor that truly excited me. I wanted to *help* my patients. Long-term health improvement seemed incomparable to just symptom relief using drugs and surgeries.

The chiropractic health model made so much sense to me that I abandoned my life-long ambition to become a medical doctor and applied instead to chiropractic school.

Once I graduated and was in my own chiropractic practice seeing real-world patients, my idealistic "the body can heal itself" ideals took a hit. I realized that chiropractic adjusting by itself wasn't resolving many of my patient's chronic health conditions. A patient would come in for an adjustment to handle their pain problem and tell me, "My doc has me scheduled for gall bladder surgery next week." I had no answer for this.

If a patient came in with symptoms of a condition beyond what chiropractic would usually help, I had no solutions. In school, we were taught that the correct action for a patient that didn't respond to chiropractic care was to refer them... to a medical doctor.

Now, with my own medical diagnosis I was in the same situation that I had been taught to put my own patients in—I was being told that the only solution to my problem was medical treatment. That fundamental, wonderful concept of the body healing itself was apparently out the window. It was drugs and surgery—or nothing (other than dire warnings of horrendous consequences).

One thing I've always excelled at is asking for information. I ask for directions if I'm lost; I collar the first store clerk I see and ask where the canned coconut milk is. So I started calling everyone I knew to find out who they might know that could help me. And I found out about Dr. Paul in Minnesota. A friend's friend's wife had once gone to Dr. Paul with a serious health condition. He knew what to do about it... and she got better. I got his number and called him.

Dr. Paul was very friendly and helpful on the phone and suggested that I pay him a visit so he could show me how he practiced.

This is how I wound up helping my husband navigate the back roads of an Indian reservation in central Minnesota. Dr. Paul had a practice in a town with a population of 200. He was a chiropractor, but also utilized half a dozen other techniques as well.

We spent two days with Dr. Paul. On the first day, I was sure I had wasted money and time to travel all the way from Atlanta into the middle of nowhere to talk to a nut case. But by the second day, I began to understand a whole new way of looking at the body, health and treatment. Dr. Paul knew more physiology and biochemistry than many of my professors at school, and he knew how to apply this information to get patients well. Dr. Paul understood that a body is an intelligent lifeform, that it communicates with itself and its environment—and that the information in this communication can be accessed and utilized to help the body to heal.

This is really the basis of acupuncture, homeopathy, chiropractic and countless other valid therapies, though I have found that often the practitioners themselves don't understand that this is true.

Dr. Paul tested me using his techniques and equipment. Everything he found made complete sense and opened the door to effective actions I could take to help my own health and healing. Finally, I had an alternative approach to drugs and surgery that I'd been looking for.

I went home and immediately started on Dr. Paul's program of diet and supplements. With some searching, I found a MD who had a slightly more open mind than my ex-doctor, so I could get lab testing done to monitor my condition. After nine months, he tested me and was amazed that my condition had not worsened. A year later, he was astonished again—I was getting better! Then I got pregnant, and after the birth was tested again... completely normal! And I have maintained this condition for twenty years to the present.

MY PATH TO DEVELOPING THE EVECTICS^{SM} HEALTH THERAPY SYSTEMS

The day I got home from my trip to the backwoods of Minnesota and Dr. Paul, I decided to completely change the way I practiced in my clinic. I saw there were techniques and methods of treatment that could be the answer for people who thought only drugs and surgeries would help with their health problems. I saw possible therapies for conditions that previously could only be managed with drugs and invasive and damaging medical procedures, or had no available treatment at all.

I decided that my clinic would become what I was looking for the day I got that terrifying phone call.

I was bursting with excitement to get started. There was only a single problem in my way: How to do this?

I informed my organizational consultant husband that he was hereby drafted into helping me, and we spent a weekend at a remote mountain cabin with papers, books and computers spread out all over analyzing the problem.

We decided on the basic requirements of the treatment process we were developing:

1. To have as an end goal a *restoration of health*, not just long- or short-term symptom improvement.

2. To achieve and maintain improved health, a patient would have to have specific, permanent lifestyle and diet improvements. People have trouble with these changes; we needed a system that would work.

3. My program must successfully address functional stresses like hormone imbalances, allergies and immune deficiencies that otherwise would stop the healing process.

4. My process must provide every patient with an *individualized* program, customized to his or her case. Also, the program must adjust and change as the patient heals.

5. My program would have to get rapid and continuing results on patients, because in my experience this is the

only way to keep a patient motivated enough to do a program to completion.

Now that I had a basic outline of what I was creating, I decided that the next step would be to attempt to learn everything that was known about this method of healing. I started jumping on airplanes at every opportunity to go to seminars and visit the practices of successful practitioners. I read constantly, watched endless video tapes and practiced the techniques I learned, mainly on my long-suffering husband. (Note: I am still just as engaged in this "learn what is known" project as I was twenty years ago; I am just no longer expecting to ever complete the job!)

After a few months of working out the basics, I changed my clinic from chiropractic-only to a nutritional practice. My fear that my patients would not take kindly to this change and whether I could keep paying my bills turned out to be unfounded—they began to heal from all kinds of problems! I was on my way to my goal!

I first changed my practice to nutritional techniques in 1996. Since that time, I have never slowed down my research efforts. Although I spend a good amount of time now on the teaching side of the podium, I still go to an endless stream of seminars, constantly make new contacts, visit practices and generally continue to polish and improve what we do at the clinic.

Several years ago, we gave what we do a name to make it easier to communicate. We call our integrated techniques and treatment programming systems "**Evectics**[SM]" (e VEK tics) an old word from the 1800s that used to mean "The branch of medical science which teaches the method of acquiring a good habit of body." Quaint, but accurate!

"Good habit of body" means that the body is well constructed and attractive. A definition of "habit" is "bodily appearance or makeup."

ABOUT THE AUTHOR

Dr. Melodie M. Billiot

Dr. Billiot is the founder and owner of Alternative Health Atlanta, Holistic Practice Solutions (a company that develops techniques and management systems for holistic practitioners) and is the developer of **Evectics**[SM] health therapy systems. She is known nationwide as an expert and sought-after teacher of nutritional and energetic techniques.

Dr. Melodie Billiot graduated from Life University in 1993 summa cum laude as valedictorian of her class. She is certified in CRA and Nutrition Response Testing, System Desensitization Technique (SDT) and N.A.E.T. allergy elimination techniques, System Balancing Technique (SBT), JMT, several chiropractic-adjusting techniques, and she has studied extensively in homeopathy, herbology, Chinese medicine, clinical nutrition and pain control using nutrition.

In 1994, she became frustrated because of a lack of consistent results with chiropractic treatment in areas other than musculoskeletal. Motivated to find a solution for her patients other than drugs and surgery and fighting a serious health problem of her own, she started researching holistic and nutritional techniques. Because of this research, Dr. Billiot recovered her own health and made significant improvements in her results with patients. Currently, Dr. Billiot has one of the most successful holistic practices in the country and trains other practitioners in clinical nutrition and other holistic techniques. She lives in Marietta, Ga with her husband, their two boys, two dogs and two cats.

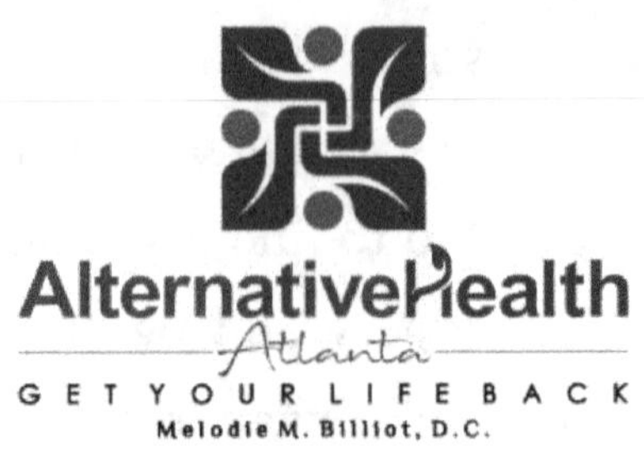

Invitation

For more information and education on hormone health problems, or to learn about treatment options with my clinic, I invite you to join me at **AlternativeHealthAtlanta.com.**

Alternative Health Atlanta

1640 Powers Ferry Rd

Building 14, Suite 100

Marietta, Georgia 30067

If you live outside of the Atlanta area:

We work with "out of town" patients every week. Using a system of phone consulting and occasional visits to Atlanta, we have successfully helped patients from many states in the US as well as from Canada, Nicaragua, Ireland, Spain and China.

(770) 612-1100 (for new patients, questions and inquiries)
(770) 937-9200 Reception Desk
Email: HealthHelp@AlternativeHealthAtlanta.com
Web: AlternativeHealthAtlanta.com

Please Leave a Review

Thank you for reading this book. I hope you enjoyed it, and are starting the process of recovering your health.

Now I'd like to ask you for a small favor. Would you kindly take a moment to leave a review on Amazon?

It would mean the world to me, and I am grateful for the time you take to write it!

Warmly,

Dr. Billiot

RESOURCES

1. Centers for Disease Control and Prevention. Chronic Diseases. The Power to Prevent.
    http://www.cdc.gov/chronicdisease/resources/publications/aag/chronic.htm

2. Centers for Disease Control and Prevention. Chronic Diseases.
    http://www.cdc.gov/chronicdisease/resources/publications/aag/chronic.htm

3. Centers for Disease Control and Prevention. MMWR 2013; 62 (44) 869- 873. [Data Source: 2010- 2012 NHIS]

4. Arthritis Foundation. Side Effects Possible with Arthritis Medications.
    http://www.arthritistoday.org/about-arthritis/types-of-arthritis/rheumatoid-arthritis/daily-life/managing-your-medications/ra-side-effects.php

5. Shaywitz, David, MD, PhD. What's Holding Back Cures? Our Collective Ignorance (And No, Not a Pharma Conspiracy).
    http://www.forbes.com/sites/davidshaywitz/2013/05/10/whats-holding-back-cures-our-collective-ignorance-and-no-not-a-pharma-conspiracy/

6. Centers for Disease Control and Prevention. National Diabetes Statistics Report, 2014. http://www.cdc.gov/diabetes/pubs/estimates14.htm

7. New York Times. Drug Makers Dial Down TV Advertising. February 2, 2012. http://prescriptions.blogs.nytimes.com/2012/02/02/drug-makers-dial-down-tv-advertising/?_php=true&_type=blogs&_r=0

8. US National Library of Medicine, National Institutes of Health. Louis Pasteur, the Father of Immunology? http://www.ncbi.nlm.nih.gov/pmc/articles/PMC3342039/

9. USA Today. Diabetes rates skyrocket in kids and teens. May, 3, 2014. http://www.usatoday.com/story/news/nation/2014/05/03/diabetes-rises-in-kids/8604213/

10. Centers for Disease Control and Prevention. Trends in Allergic Conditions Among Children: US, 1997-2011. http://www.cdc.gov/nchs/data/databriefs/db121.pdf

11. Centers for Disease Control and Prevention. Developmental Disabilities. Key Findings: Trends in the Prevalence of Developmental Disabilities in US Children, 1977-2008. http://www.cdc.gov/ncbddd/developmentaldisabilities/features/birthdefects-dd-keyfindings.html